W9-DFE-224

Vaccines

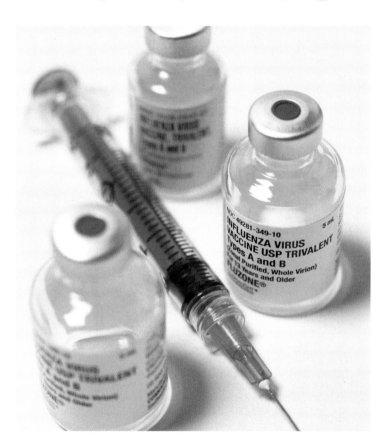

Carol Ellis

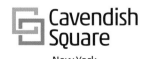

Cavendish
Square

New York

Published in 2014 by Cavendish Square Publishing, LLC
303 Park Avenue South, Suite 1247, New York, NY 10010

Copyright © 2014 by Cavendish Square Publishing, LLC

First Edition

Website: cavendishsq.com

This publication represents the opinions and views of the author based on his or her personal experience, knowledge, and research. The information in this book serves as a general guide only. The author and publisher have used their best efforts in preparing this book and disclaim liability rising directly or indirectly from the use and application of this book.

CPSIA Compliance Information: Batch #WS13CSQ

All websites were available and accurate when this book was sent to press.

Library of Congress Cataloging-in-Publication Data
Ellis, Carol.
Vaccines / Carol Ellis.
p. cm. — (Advances in medicine)
Includes bibliographical references and index.
Summary: "Discusses the advances that have been made in vaccinations"—Provided by publisher.
ISBN 978-1-60870-470-5 (hardcover) ISBN 978-1-62712-012-8 (paperback) ISBN 978-1-60870-597-9 (ebook)
1. Vaccines—Juvenile literature. I. Title. II. Series.
RM281.E45 2012
615'.372—dc22
2010044011

Editors: Megan Comerford / Joyce Stanton / Christine Florie
Art Director: Anahid Hamparian   Series Designer: Nancy Sabato

Photo research by Edward Thomas

The photographs in this book are used by permission and through the courtesy of: *Cutcaster*: ArenaCreative, Back Cover & Openers; *Getty Images*: Peter Ardito/Photolibrary, 1; David C Tomlinson, 7; Jose Luis Pelaez, 8; Joe Raedle, 37; Chris Hondros, 52, Charles Dharapak, 53; *The Image Works*: ©NMPFT/Daily Herald Archive/SSPL, 4; *Superstock*: © BSIP, 9; © Bridgeman Art Library, 21; © Blend Images, 40; © Science Faction, 43; *Photo Researchers, Inc.*: SPL, 11, 32; 3D4Medical, 25; Saturn Stills, 35; *The Bridgeman Art Library International*: Edward Jenner (1749-1823) performing the first vaccination against Smallpox in 1796, 1879 (oil on canvas) (detail) (see also 166614), Melingue, Gaston (1840-1914) / Academie Nationale de Medecine, Paris, France / Archives Charmet, 14; Plaque depicting 'The Origin of Vaccination', late 18th century (glazed ceramic), French School, (18th century) / Private Collection / Archives Charmet, 17; *Alamy*: © INTERFOTO, 22; © Everett Collection Inc., 27, 28; *Newscom*: Agencia Fotolia/El Tiempo de Colombia, 44; *AP Images*: Greg Campbell, 48.

Printed in the United States of America

contents

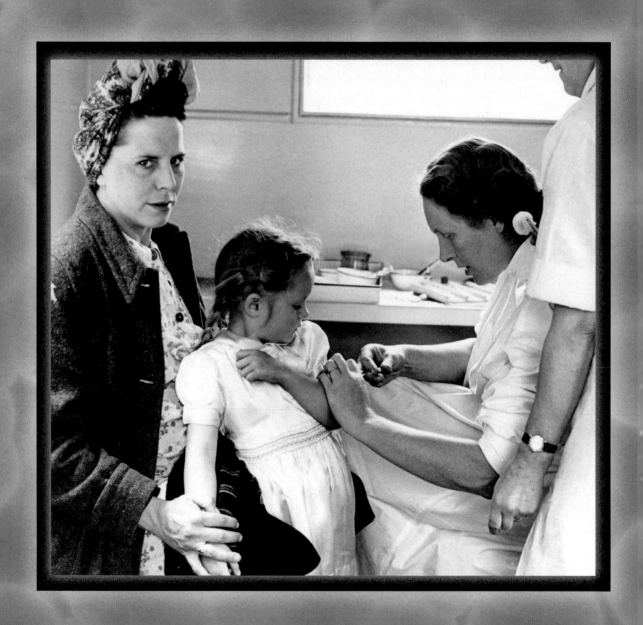

chapter 1

What Are Vaccines?

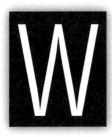**W**hen Lily was three years old, she developed a sore throat and a fever. The glands in her neck grew swollen, and it was difficult for her to swallow. She began to have trouble breathing because of a thick, grayish black membrane that covered part of her throat like a piece of duct tape. The membrane was a telltale sign: Lily had **diphtheria**. Just the word sent shivers of fear throughout neighborhoods

A young girl receives a vaccine for diphtheria in 1949.
Prior to immunizations, many children died from this disease.

and communities. Diphtheria is highly **contagious**. It can kill. It strikes mostly young children. When Lucy had diphtheria, there was no cure.

Lily had diphtheria during the early 1920s, a time when the United States saw approximately 150,000 cases and 13,000 deaths from this bacterial infection. Lily survived, but the disease had already done its damage. Even though she lived for many more years, her heart remained weakened for the rest of her life.

When Lily's daughter Barbara was six years old, she, too, survived a disease that affected mostly children. It started like a common cold with a cough. After about a week, the cough got worse. Terrible coughing spells went on for almost three weeks. They were so violent that Barbara vomited and her face turned purple. She couldn't catch her breath. When she was finally able to breathe air into her lungs, she made a horrible whooping sound. She had **pertussis**, or whooping cough. Like diphtheria, pertussis is caused by **bacteria**. It is spread by coughing and sneezing, and is very contagious. During the 1940s, when Barbara had it, it was a major cause of death in children. Barbara recovered. But even after the coughing spells ended, it took another month before she felt completely well.

The illness Barbara's daughter Sarah remembers best from her childhood is **chicken pox**. Most of her friends had it when they were five or six years old. It was no fun, but it wasn't a big deal. Sarah's friends were itchy and uncomfortable for about a week. Then they got over it. But for Sarah the story was different. Sarah didn't get chicken pox until she was fourteen. For her the disease was a lot more severe.

Chicken pox, a disease caused by a **virus**, produces a red, itchy skin rash. The rash starts out as little bumps and then develops into fluid-filled blisters.

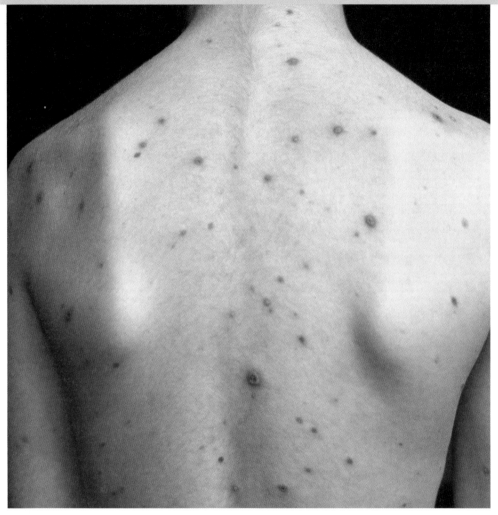

The chicken pox virus causes red, itchy blisters. The chicken pox vaccine fights off this virus.

In Sarah's case, those blisters spread over most parts of her body. She even had them inside her mouth. Her mom did everything she could to help ease the maddening itch: lukewarm oatmeal baths; cool, wet compresses; soft mittens at night so Barbara couldn't scratch the blisters in her sleep. On top of everything else, Sarah developed **pneumonia** and had to go to the hospital. Her doctor said that this sometimes happens when teenagers and adults get chicken pox. Sarah recovered from both the chicken pox and the pneumonia, but to this day she won't eat pudding!

Abby is just about ready to enter middle school. She is Sarah's daughter, and she has heard all about her mother's chicken pox. She knows about her grandmother's whooping cough, too, and her great-grandmother's diphtheria. Abby has never had those or many other diseases. The chances are very good that she never will. In the years since her great-grandmother was sick, scientists have developed vaccines that help prevent people from getting certain diseases.

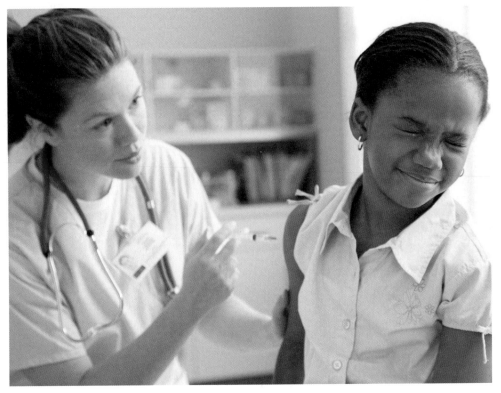

Today, there are vaccinations that prevent people from contracting serious illnesses.

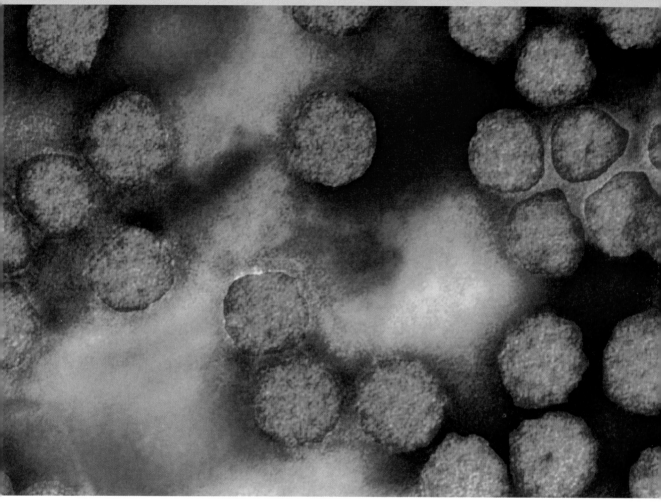

This is an image of the German measles virus as seen through a high-powered microscope.

Battling Foreign Invaders

Vaccines help your body fight off invasions from bacteria and viruses that cause disease. Bacteria and viruses are microbes—organisms that are too small to see without the help of a microscope. Bacteria are made up of only one cell. Viruses are even smaller.

You come into contact with millions of microbes every day. Not all of them are harmful. Some are even helpful, such as the bacteria that live in your digestive tract. But some microbes that get into your body can give you a serious disease or even cause your death. That's where vaccines come in.

Vaccines work within your immune system—a network of cells, glands, organs, and fluids. If you think of your body as a fortress, then the immune system is a finely organized troop of soldiers constantly on the alert for invading enemies. One of those enemies is the **measles** virus.

Picture yourself growing up during the 1950s. You were on a school bus, and another student had the measles but didn't know it yet. When your seatmate coughed and sneezed, tiny droplets containing hundreds of measles viruses spread through the air. You breathed them in. Once inside your body, the viruses set about replicating, or making copies of themselves. The hundreds of viruses soon became millions.

However, all of those viruses quickly ran into your immune system's first line of defense—special white blood cells called **macrophages**, which means "big eaters." The white blood cells could tell that the viruses were invaders because they had markers called **antigens**—molecules that identified them as "foreign." The microphages grabbed onto as many of the viruses as they could and chewed them up. But they saved the antigens and carried them back to other areas in the immune system. There, they showed the antigens to other white blood cells—the T cells and B cells. These cells immediately went into action.

Meanwhile, you developed the first signs that your immune system was fighting an infection. You had a runny nose, a dry cough, and a fever.

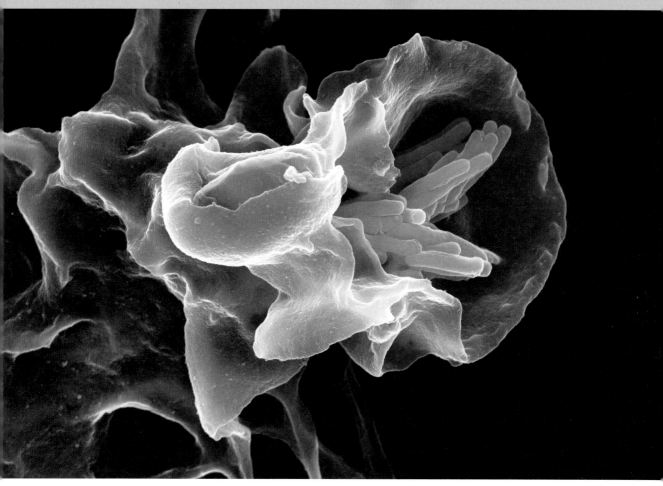

An electron microscope captures a macrophage engulfing a tuberculosis bacterium (green).

Back inside your body, the war escalated. "Killer" T cells secreted, or released, chemicals. Those chemicals destroyed many of your cells that had already been invaded by the measles virus. The B cells made weapons called **antibodies**. In fact, the B cells manufacture millions of antibodies that circulate in your blood all the time. Each antibody has to conform to the special shape of an antigen. In this case it was the antigen of the measles virus.

When the antibodies came across the measles antigens lurking in your system, they latched onto them and signaled the big eaters—the macrophages—to come destroy them.

By this time you knew you had the measles. It started with tiny white spots with bluish centers on the inside of your mouth and cheeks. Then a reddish brown rash appeared on your forehead and behind your ears. The blotchy rash spread down to cover your trunk, arms, and legs. Your fever rose to 104 degrees Fahrenheit. On top of that, you developed a painful ear infection—a side effect that sometimes occurs with the measles. You felt absolutely rotten.

Your immune system kept up the battle for almost two weeks. Finally it got the better of the measles virus. The T cells and antibodies were able to destroy the virus faster than it could replicate. The rash began to fade. You began to feel better. Soon you went back to your normal life and forgot about the measles.

But your immune system did not forget. After the B cells and T cells helped get rid of the virus, some of them converted into memory cells. They would circulate through your body for the rest of your life. If the measles virus were ever to invade again, those cells would be able to destroy it so fast you wouldn't even realize it was there. You had become immune to the measles. Becoming immune to a disease by catching it and getting over it is called naturally acquired immunity.

Fast-forward twenty years, to the 1970s. Scientists have developed a measles vaccine, and you have been vaccinated. The vaccine mimics a natural measles infection, but with a big difference: you don't get sick. The vaccine contains an **attenuated**, or weakened, version of the virus. It can't cause a fever, cough, rash, or any side effects such as an ear infection or pneumonia. But the vaccine antigens are strong enough to trick your immune system into thinking it is under attack. It goes into action. The macrophages, T cells, and B cells behave just as they would if you had actually been infected with the natural measles virus. They clear up the mock infection quickly. They also create memory cells to protect you if you're ever exposed to measles in the future. The vaccine, not the virus itself, has made you immune. Getting vaccinated had given you artificially acquired immunity.

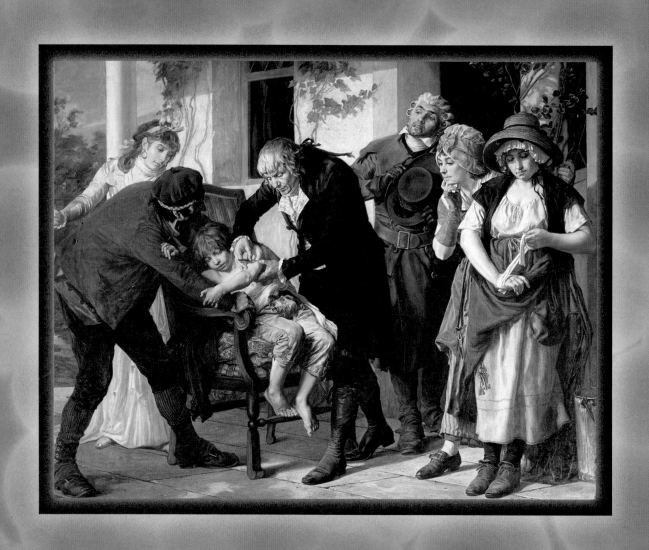

chapter 2

History of Vaccines

In the summer of 1796, an English country doctor named Edward Jenner made a few scratches on the arm of eight-year-old James Phipps. He then smeared some pus from a cowpox blister into the scratches. Cowpox was a mild skin disease transmitted from cows to humans, most often farmworkers. Sure enough, James developed cowpox. He recovered quickly. A few weeks later, Doctor Jenner got to the heart of his experiment: he infected James with pus from a **smallpox** blister. Like cowpox, smallpox is caused by a virus. In fact, it's from the same family of viruses as cowpox. But unlike cowpox, smallpox isn't mild. It is deadly.

Doctor Edward Jenner performs the first vaccination against smallpox.

Smallpox had been around for thousands of years. Many scholars believe that scars on the mummy of Egyptian pharaoh Ramses V were caused by smallpox. Smallpox was such a major killer of infants that some people were afraid to name a newborn until it got the disease and survived. Explorers carried the virus to the Americas, where it devastated the Aztecs, Incas, and tribes of North American Indians. Every year during the eighteenth century, smallpox epidemics in Europe killed an estimated 400,000 people. The disease killed one out of every ten children born in Sweden and France and one out of every seven children born in Russia.

Smallpox begins suddenly, with high fever, chills, and intense shivering. Then comes the rash, which turns into blisters on the face, inside the eyes, and then over the entire body. Eventually, the blisters harden and the scabs fall off, leaving deep, pitted scars. Those who survived smallpox were disfigured for life. Many were left blind.

During Jenner's time, many people believed that if they got cowpox, they wouldn't get smallpox. In fact, a milkmaid told Jenner that because she'd had cowpox, she would never have to live with a scarred and pitted face. No one knew why having a cowpox infection seemed to protect them from smallpox. Jenner didn't know why either, but he wanted to find out. This led to his experiment with James Phipps. It was risky. After all, Jenner was deliberately infecting someone with smallpox. But James did not develop the disease. Jenner exposed him to it several more times, but James never came down with smallpox. Jenner had created a way to make people immune to smallpox. He had created a vaccine.

While Jenner was not the first person to try this experiment, he was the first one who was able to show and convince people that getting a vaccination would work. He didn't know how the immune system functioned. He didn't know about antigens and antibodies, microphages, and memory cells. If he had, he would have said that the antigens of cowpox were similar enough to the antigens of smallpox that the body's immune system recognized the smallpox antigens as enemies and produced antibodies to fight them.

Because the substance Jenner used in his experiment came from a cowpox blister, he called his discovery a vaccine, from *vacca*, the Latin word for "cow." The word would stick and eventually be used for all vaccines, no matter where they came from. And although Jenner didn't live to see it, his technique of vaccination eventually helped the body defend itself against many other diseases, such as diphtheria, measles, **polio**, and **rabies**.

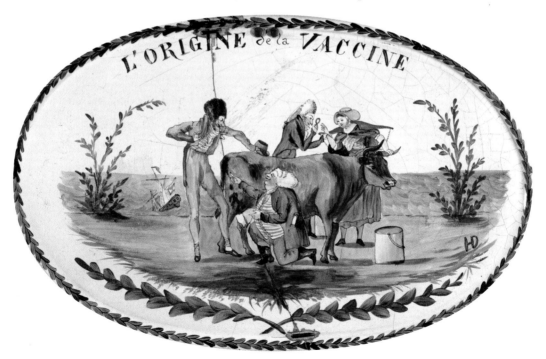

A French plaque from the late 1700s depicts the origins of vaccinations.

A LONG ROAD TO PREVENTION

People had tried to combat smallpox for thousands of years. One thing everyone knew was that if you got smallpox and recovered, you would not get it again. This led to the idea of deliberately infecting people with matter taken from smallpox blisters. The idea was that they would get a mild form of the disease, recover, and be safe for the rest of their lives. The process was called "variolation." Sometimes dried smallpox scabs would be ground into powder and blown into someone's nostrils. Another method was to insert the smallpox matter under the skin. Variolation was often used in China, India, and Turkey.

By the 1700s the technique had spread to Europe. Jenner himself was variolated when he was a child. It was a terrible experience. Six weeks of preparation included his being bled and made to fast until he was very thin. Then he was finally infected with smallpox. He did not have a mild case, but he survived. Many did. Many others did not. Even those who did survive were contagious while they had it. They could spread the disease to others and make an epidemic even worse. As a solution to smallpox, variolation did not work. Jenner found a solution that *did* work: vaccination.

Pasteur, Germs, and Disease

By the middle of the 1800s, vaccination was common for smallpox, but not for any other disease. The medical world still did not fully understand how the vaccine worked, and the human immune system was still a mystery. Louis Pasteur, a French scientist, took the study and technology of vaccines a giant step further. His research into vaccines began with animals.

In 1879 the barnyards of France were under siege. A bacterial disease called chicken cholera was killing nine out of every ten chickens it infected. The epidemic threatened the livelihoods of thousands of poultry farmers.

Pasteur set about trying to find a way to produce a vaccine. He found it almost by accident. He took samples of the chicken cholera bacteria and grew them in cultures in his laboratory. One day, after returning from a summer vacation, he discovered that his assistants had left the cultures out in the heat. Instead of throwing the cultures away, he tested them on healthy chickens. The batch of cholera bacteria gave them only a mild case of the disease. When he injected them with fresh bacteria, they did not become sick at all. The heat had weakened the bacteria. The vaccine was too weak to kill the chickens, but it was strong enough to teach their immune systems how to protect them from further infection. The chickens were now immune to the cholera.

Pasteur knew about Jenner's work with smallpox eighty years earlier. In that case, the germs from a different, milder disease had protected the body from a stronger one. Pasteur had discovered a method of weakening the germs of a disease and using them in a vaccine to combat the same disease.

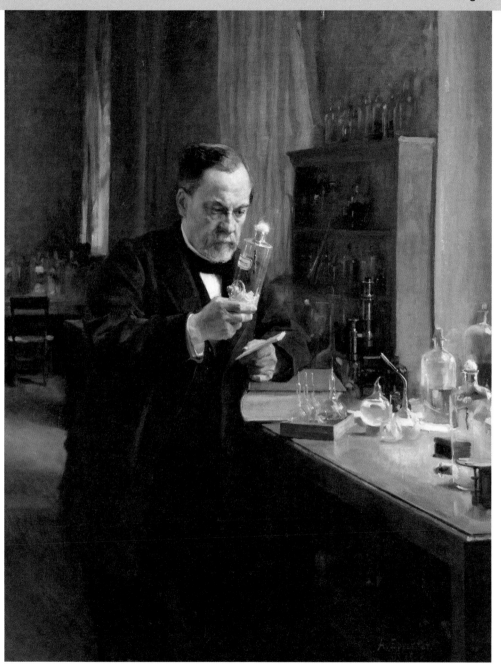

French scientist Louis Pasteur developed vaccines for several diseases, including rabies.

Pasteur next turned his focus to **anthrax**. Anthrax is a fatal disease that affects sheep, cattle, and sometimes humans. Thanks to the work of the German scientist Robert Koch, Pasteur and others knew that a bacterium caused the disease.

As he had done with the chicken cholera bacteria, Pasteur grew the anthrax bacteria in his lab. After many experiments, he was able to weaken the bacteria by exposing it to air and aging it over time. His announcement of a vaccine caused a lot of excitement as well as some disbelief. A well-known veterinarian was so skeptical that he challenged Pasteur. To prove that the vaccine would work, he demanded that Pasteur perform a carefully controlled test in public. Pasteur accepted the challenge. The test took

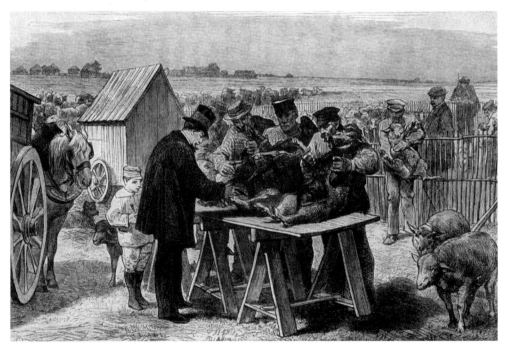

Louis Pasteur vaccinates sheep against anthrax, dramatically confirming his vaccine.

THE GERM THEORY

"I am afraid that the experiments you quote, Monsieur Pasteur, will turn against you. The world into which you wish to take us is really too fantastic." So said many in the medical profession when Pasteur claimed that tiny, airborne **microorganisms**, commonly called germs, caused beer, wine, and milk to go sour. He did not pay attention to the ridicule. He kept on experimenting. Eventually Pasteur was able to convince most people that infectious diseases in humans were also caused by microorganisms. This came to be known as the germ theory of disease.

Pasteur developed a way to make milk, cheese, and other foods safe from germs by heating the food to destroy the harmful microorganisms. Today "pasteurization" is widely used to preserve food. Thanks to Pasteur's germ theory, hospitals are kept as clean and germfree as possible, and the "fantastic" world of **microbiology** has become a science.

place in 1881 on a farm outside Paris. Twenty-five sheep were vaccinated and twenty-five were not. Then all were deliberately injected with anthrax. The twenty-five vaccinated sheep remained healthy. The twenty-five unvaccinated sheep died.

The next animal vaccine Pasteur developed was for rabies, a viral disease that attacks the central nervous system. He had tested his vaccine on dogs, with promising results. Then, in 1885, nine-year-old Joseph Meister and his mother turned up at Pasteur's laboratory. Joseph had been badly mauled by a rabid dog two days earlier. Testing his vaccine on a human was risky, and Pasteur was reluctant to do it. But Joseph would most likely die, since rabies is nearly always fatal once the symptoms appear. So Pasteur took the chance. It turned out that his vaccine, which immunized dogs, was able to stop the rabies virus before it could invade Joseph's brain and spinal cord. Joseph never developed the disease.

After Pasteur's success with rabies, the development of vaccines for humans grew quickly. Improved techniques and new technology helped scientists learn much more about microbes and the workings of the immune system. The electron microscope, invented in 1931, let them see viruses for the first time. Vaccines for deadly diseases such as diphtheria, pertussis, and **tetanus** were developed by the 1940s.

Salk, Sabin, and the Polio Vaccine

The polio virus is five thousand times smaller than the width of a human hair. In the early 1950s people in the United States were terrified of it. Polio outbreaks were not new. Epidemics had occurred in the country every

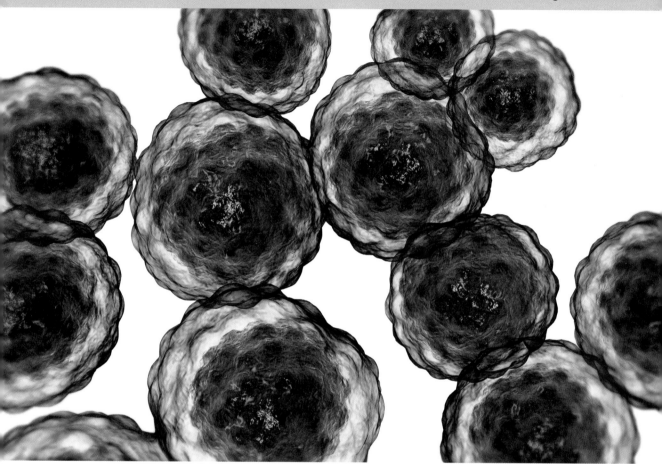

A microscopic view of the polio virus.

year since 1916. But 1952 was the worst. About 600,000 cases were reported worldwide that year. Almost 60,000 of them were in the United States.

The polio virus usually caused only flulike symptoms. Ninety-five percent of people recovered without a problem. However, for the other 5 percent, the virus could be fatal. It invades a victim's central nervous system and destroys the motor neuron cells. Motor neurons control the muscles for swallowing, circulation, and breathing. At its worst, polio causes **paralysis** or even death, especially when it paralyzes the muscles that are needed to breathe. Hospital wards filled with children lying in "iron lungs," mechanical devices that breathed for them. Thousands of children left the hospital in wheelchairs. Polio affects only humans, and there is no cure for it.

Because polio usually struck during the summer and early fall, people often talked of "polio weather." Parents kept their kids out of public swimming pools and away from large public gatherings. They insisted on frequent hand washing. One woman remembers a friend not being allowed to eat peaches during the summer because of the belief that the virus might thrive on peach fuzz. A man who survived polio remembers that he was not allowed to see his parents except through a hospital window. When he finally went home, he had to leave behind the toy truck that his parents had given him. Polio was highly contagious. Everything the patients had handled was burned.

Most of polio's victims were children. But it affected people of all ages. President Franklin D. Roosevelt was paralyzed by the disease when he was thirty-nine. After he took office, he promoted research for a vaccine. This led to the development of an organization called the March of Dimes. Schools, businesses, churches, and other groups collected dimes for research to help find a way to fight polio. With some of the money, the March of Dimes hired a researcher named Jonas Salk.

Doctor Salk had been doing research on polio for several years. He was sure that he could find a safe vaccine. By the height of the epidemic, in 1952, he had developed one. Testing began in 1954. People were so afraid of polio

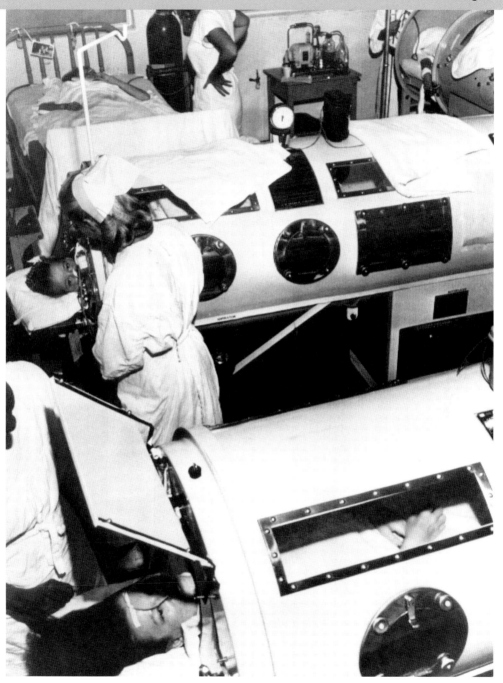

Polio patients being treated with iron lungs in 1948.

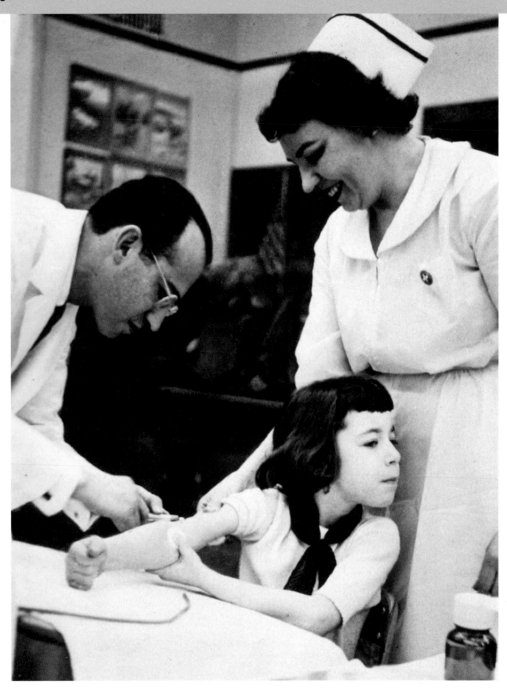

Doctor Jonas Salk inoculates a child with the polio vaccine, now known as the Salk vaccine.

that they did not have to be persuaded to volunteer for the test. Almost 2 million children around the country lined up for shots. Some of them received the vaccine, others received a placebo, a shot that did not contain the vaccine. All of them got a piece of candy and an official card that declared them to be Polio Pioneers.

The results of the test were announced over the radio in 1955. The vaccine was a success. People cheered as if their favorite baseball team had won the World Series.

Meanwhile, another researcher in the United States, Albert Sabin, developed a second type of polio vaccine that could be given by mouth instead of by injection. Because Salk's vaccine was already being used in the United States, Sabin tested his in the Soviet Union. This was during the cold war, but people were too afraid of polio to let politics get in the way. In 1959, ten million children in the Soviet Union received the vaccine. The program was a success. Albert Sabin received a medal of gratitude from the Russian government.

Today, the Salk vaccine is used mostly in the United States and Europe. The Sabin vaccine is used in other areas of the world.

Vaccine Success Stories

Advances came even more quickly in the second half of the twentieth century and in the first decade of the twenty-first. In the United States, the effect of vaccines was dramatic for a number of diseases:

- Before the diphtheria vaccine (1930s), there were between 100,000 and 200,000 cases and about 14,000 deaths a year. Today there are about 2 or 3 cases a year.

- Between 3 million and 4 million cases of measles occurred every year before a vaccine became available in 1963. After that, measles infections were reduced by 98 percent.
- About 250,000 cases of **mumps** occurred every year until a vaccine became available in the 1960s. Today only about 250 cases occur each year.
- From 1964 to 1965 there were 20,000 cases of **rubella** (German measles). The viral disease caused 11,000 children to be born deaf, 3,500 to be born blind, and 1,800 to be born intellectually disabled. Since a vaccine has come into use, only 5 or 6 cases are reported each year.
- Polio paralyzed more than 21,000 people in 1952. Most of them were children. A vaccine came into use a few years later. Since 1979 there have been no more cases of "wild" polio—polio that occurs naturally—in the United States.
- Tetanus is a disease caused by a toxin, or poison, produced by a bacterium. It is also known as lockjaw because paralysis starts in the jaw and moves down the body. About 11 percent of cases are fatal. Tetanus is not passed from person to person. It usually enters the body through a wound. The bacteria thrive in soil and cannot be destroyed. Between 1922 and 1926 there were approximately 1,300 cases of tetanus in the United States. A vaccine came into use in the late 1940s. Between 2001 and 2005, only 142 cases of tetanus were reported in the United States.
- In 1980 the World Health Organization (WHO) announced that smallpox had been completely wiped out, not just in the United States but around the world. If you were born after that date, you did not have to get the smallpox vaccine. A disease that had plagued the world for centuries was no longer a threat.

Vaccine-Preventable Diseases 2010

Disease	Date Vaccine Discovered or Licensed for Use
Anthrax, for humans	1970
Bacterial meningitis	1970, 2005 (two types of vaccines)
Cervical cancer	2006
Chicken pox	1995
Diphtheria	1923
Hepatitis A	1995
Hepatitis B	1982
Hib disease	1990
Influenza	1940s
Japanese encephalitis	1993
Measles	1963
Mumps	1967
Pertussis	1926
Pneumococcal disease	1977
Polio	1955
Rabies	1885
Rotavirus diarrhea	1998
Rubella	1969
Shingles	2006
Smallpox	1798
Tetanus	1927
Tuberculosis	1927
Typhoid	1990
Yellow Fever	1930

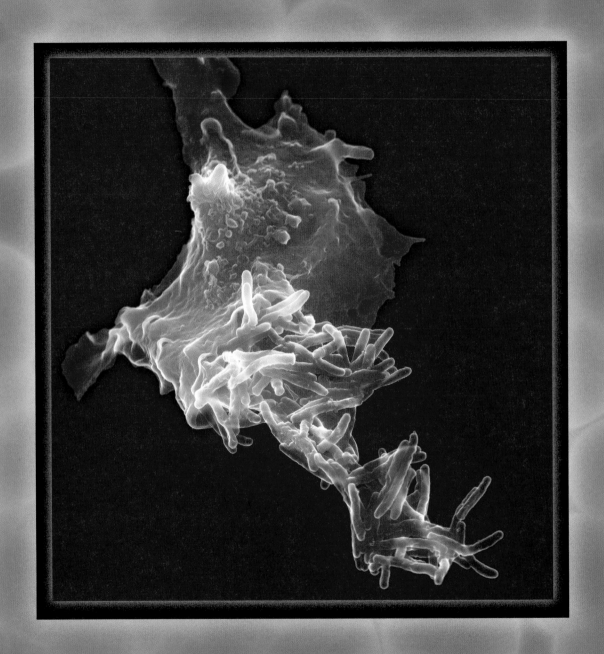

chapter 3

How Are Vaccines Made?

The goal of a vaccine is to trick your immune system into thinking it is under attack so that it will fight off the mock infection and create memory cells that will give you immunity to a natural infection. Since a vaccine contains the disease-causing microbes, the trick is to keep the vaccine itself from giving you any symptoms of the disease. To do this, scientists use different methods to create different kinds of vaccines.

A colored scan shows a macrophage white blood cell (red) attacking a live, but weakened, strain of tuberculosis bacteria from a vaccine.

Attenuated Vaccines

Live, attenuated vaccines contain a weakened version of the living microbe. In the lab, the microbe is passed through cell cultures many times. This weakens it to the point where it can't cause serious disease, but it will still get the immune system to create antibodies and memory cells. Live vaccines work especially well for viruses. A natural virus reproduces itself thousands of times. A weakened vaccine virus usually reproduces itself only about twenty times, so the immune system has almost no trouble getting rid of it.

Since a live but weak vaccine is the closest thing to a natural infection, it's a great "teacher" of the immune system. One or two doses of this type of vaccine often give a person lifetime immunity. Vaccines for measles, mumps, rubella, and chicken pox are examples of live vaccines. Albert Sabin's polio oral vaccine is a live, weakened vaccine.

Live vaccines, however, have a couple of drawbacks. Even though the microbe has been weakened, it is still a living organism. It is unlikely but possible that it could mutate, or change, into a dangerous form. Then it could cause infection. A second drawback is that live vaccines can't be given to people whose immune systems are weakened, such as from chemotherapy or HIV/AIDS.

Inactivated Vaccines

Inactivated vaccines are vaccines in which the microbe has been killed with chemicals, heat, or a type of **radiation**. However, the body still detects it, so the immune system produces antibodies to protect itself. The rabies, flu, and **hepatitis A** vaccines are made this way. Jonas Salk's polio vaccine is, too.

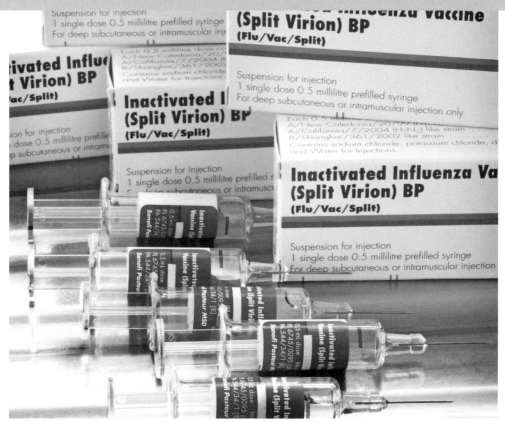

Inactivated influenza vaccines stimulate the body's immune system to produce antibodies without causing infection.

Inactivated vaccines are safer than live ones because a dead microbe cannot reproduce and cause infection. People with weakened immune systems can get this type of vaccine. And unlike most live vaccines, inactivated vaccines do not need to be refrigerated. This makes it easy to store and transport them.

The disadvantage to an inactivated vaccine is that the immune system does not respond to it as strongly as it does to a live vaccine. Several doses are needed before someone is completely immune to the disease. That means receiving booster shots!

FIGHTING THE FLU

For a lot of people, getting **influenza**, or the flu, means a couple of weeks of aches, fever, and feeling miserable. For a lot of others, though, it can be much more serious. It can even be fatal.

In 1918 the world went through one of the worst flu epidemics in history. An estimated 50 million people died. Today there are vaccines that help prevent the flu. But the virus that causes the disease is tricky. It changes from year to year. Catching the flu one year will not make you immune to next year's strain. Vaccines are up against the same problem. To keep up with the virus, the vaccine must change as well. Doctors and scientists around the world study the different strains that are circulating each year. They try to predict which ones will hit during the next flu season. Then they make a vaccine that mixes the three most likely strains.

Two types of vaccines can be used to protect people from the flu. One is an inactivated vaccine. It is usually given by injection in the arm. The second, a mist that is sprayed into the nose, is a live, weakened vaccine. The flu shot is recommended for people ages six months or older. The nasal spray is recommended for people ages two to forty-nine. However, since the spray contains a weak but live version of the virus, it should not be given to people with asthma, chronic heart disease, or weakened immune systems.

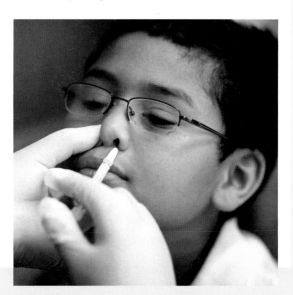

Subunit Vaccines

Subunit vaccines are made with parts of a microbe instead of the whole thing. In the case of a virus, the vaccine is made from a protein on the virus's surface. The **hepatitis B** vaccine is made this way. It appears to give longtime immunity after three doses. It can also be given to people with weakened immune systems.

A subunit vaccine for a bacterial disease contains only the antigens that get the strongest response from the immune system. Once scientists have identified those antigens, they use chemicals to break apart the bacteria and then gather the antigens they want to use.

A special type of subunit vaccine is known as the conjugate vaccine. Many bacteria have an outer coating of sugar molecules. These molecules disguise the bacteria's antigens from the immature immune systems of infants and young children. A conjugate vaccine uses an antigen from a microbe that a young immune system can recognize. When the antigen is linked to the sugar coating of the harmful bacteria, the immune system defends itself against both. The vaccine for **Hib disease** is a conjugate vaccine.

Toxoid Vaccines

Toxoid vaccines are made from toxins secreted by some bacteria. Scientists use a mixture of formaldehyde and sterilized water to deactivate the toxin. When a toxin is deactivated, it is called a toxoid, and it can't do any damage. When a toxoid is used in a vaccine, the immune system doesn't know it is harmless, so it produces antibodies to block it. The vaccines for diphtheria and tetanus are toxoid vaccines. These types of vaccines often need booster doses after several years.

Ingredients in Vaccines

Vaccines contain other ingredients in addition to elements of the virus or bacterium:

- **Adjuvants**: Adjuvants improve the body's immune response to a vaccine. They can do this in several ways: they can bind to the antigens in the vaccine, help keep them at the site of the injection, and help deliver them to the lymph nodes, where the immune response begins. The only adjuvant currently approved for use in the United States is made of aluminum salts.
- **Antibiotics**: Antibiotics stop the growth of bacteria and are used to keep vaccines uncontaminated when being manufactured.
- **Preservatives**: Preservatives keep multidose vials of a vaccine sterile after they are opened. Before the use of preservatives, doctors might put opened portions of vaccines back in the refrigerator to keep them fresh, but bacteria would often enter the vials anyway.
- **Stabilizers**: Stabilizers are added to a vaccine to keep the ingredients from degrading, or losing their effect, during manufacture, transport, and storage. Gelatin is used as a stabilizer.

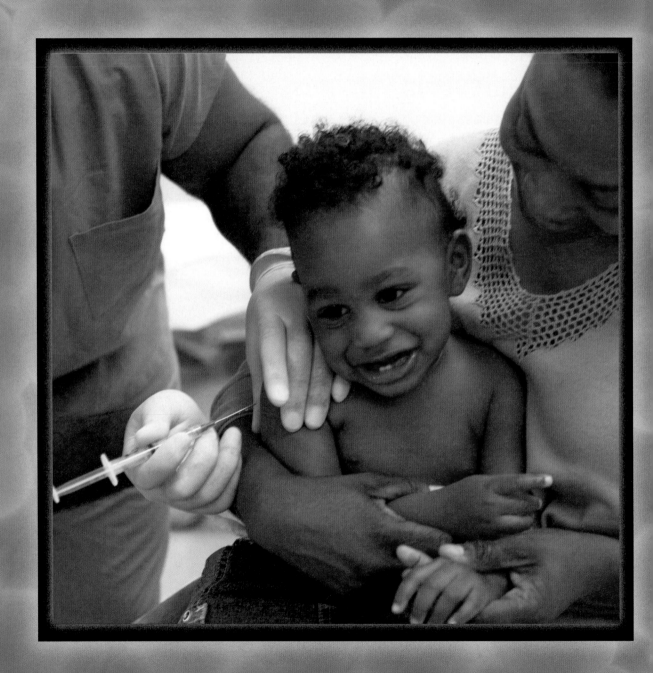

chapter 4

Vaccines: Pros, Cons, and Controversies

Since vaccines came into widespread use in the 1950s and 1960s, they have helped prevent people from contracting dozens of infectious diseases that cause serious illness or death. Many vaccines are now given to children during the first two years of life, because diseases often hit small children the hardest. In the United States and many other countries, most people are fortunate not to have to worry

Small children are given vaccines from birth to age two to ward off serious diseases.

any longer about such life-threatening illnesses as diphtheria, polio, and mumps. Smallpox is a thing of the past all over the world.

Recommended Vaccines

The following vaccines are recommended for all children, adolescents, and adults in the United States:

diphtheria	mumps
hepatitis A	pertussis (whooping cough)
hepatitis Brindlebeam	**pneumococcal disease**
Hib	polio
human papillomavirus	**rotavirus**
influenza	rubella (German measles)
measles	tetanus
meningococcus (meningitis)	varicella (chicken pox)

Pros

Vaccines have provided the world with many benefits:

- Before vaccines, the only way you could obtain immunity from a disease was to get the disease and get over it.
- Even if you got over a disease, it could leave you with lifelong disabilities. Measles can cause encephalitis, an inflammation of the brain. Mumps can cause deafness. Polio can cause paralysis.
- It is easier to prevent a disease than to treat it. Getting a vaccination is cheaper than several doctor visits or a possible stay in the hospital. And why get sick if you don't have to?

- Vaccines don't protect only you; they protect the people around you. If you've been vaccinated, you can't infect your family or friends, and vice versa. When many people in a community are immunized, fewer people can spread or catch a disease. When an entire community of people, or animals, is immune to a particular disease, it is said that they have "herd immunity."

- If you can't be vaccinated because of cancer treatments, a weak immune system, or a severe allergy to a vaccine ingredient, you are still better protected from disease if the people around you are immunized.

- Vaccines are widely available in the United States and in many other countries.

Cons

Vaccines are not perfect:

- Because new diseases, or new strains of the wily flu virus, can appear, it's not likely that vaccines will be able to help wipe out every contagious disease.

- A vaccine's trip from a lab to your doctor's office can take decades.

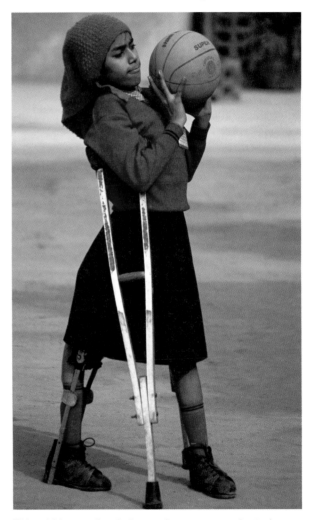

This girl is a polio victim, and was not vaccinated against the disease.

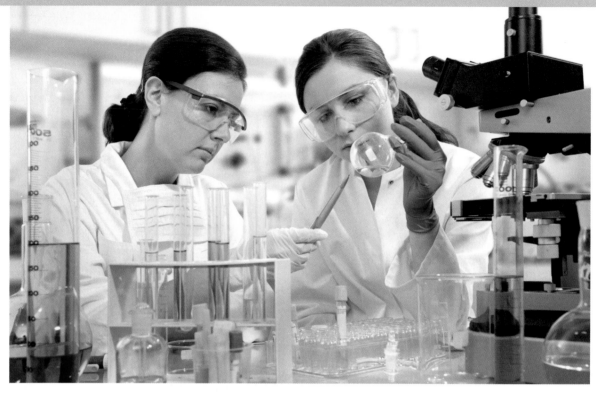

It can take researchers years to develop effective vaccinations.

First, it has to be researched and developed. Then it has to be tested. The first tests are usually on animals. Next, it has to be tested on a small number of people who volunteer to be part of the vaccine trial. After the results are known, a larger group of volunteers gets the test vaccine, and then an even larger group, this time in the tens of thousands. If those results are good, the U.S. Food and Drug Administration (FDA) will approve a license allowing the vaccine to be used in the general public.

· Many vaccines need to be refrigerated. This is easy in a country such as the United States, where goods are transported under refrigeration and everyone has electricity. It is not so easy in the remote areas of undeveloped countries.

- Vaccines don't provide 100 percent immunity to everyone. If it were possible to vaccinate every person in the world, a small percentage of them would still not have immunity. Everyone's immune system is different. A few people will not respond to a vaccine.

- Some vaccines lose their strength over time. Pertussis has been on the rise in the United States since the 1980s, especially in adolescents. One reason is that the immunity produced by the vaccine fades after five to ten years. To protect themselves and the people around them, especially infants, adolescents as well as adults should receive booster vaccines.

- Vaccines can have side effects. Most of them are not serious: a sore arm from the injection or a low fever. But some people can have serious reactions to a vaccine. For example, if a person is severely allergic to eggs, a vaccine grown in egg cultures could cause a life-threatening breathing problem.

Controversies

Can a vaccine cause the very disease it is supposed to prevent? Why should the government be allowed to require me to get vaccinated? Can a vaccine or an ingredient in a vaccine, cause another, worse disease?

Controversies and doubts about vaccines are nothing new. People have been voicing concerns about them ever since Edward Jenner developed the vaccine for smallpox.

- **Can a vaccine cause the disease it is trying to prevent?** Only a live, attenuated vaccine could do this. However, if it happened, it would almost always be a much milder form of the disease.

- **What about personal freedom and choice?** In the United States, all fifty states require children to be vaccinated against certain diseases before they start school. But many states let parents opt out of this because of religious or philosophical beliefs.

- **If there aren't many cases of a disease anymore, why bother getting vaccinated?** Smallpox is the only disease that has been eradicated from the world. Polio no longer exists in some countries, but it is definitely still out there. Other infectious diseases are, too. More people than ever travel around the world today. That makes it easier to spread the germs that cause disease.

- **Can vaccines cause other diseases or disorders?** This is one of the possibilities that has worried people the most. In the 1990s, a vaccine preservative called thimerosal was suspected of causing autism in very young children. Autism is a developmental disorder that affects a person's communication skills, social development, and behavior. The MMR (measles, mumps, rubella) vaccine was also suspected of causing autism, although it did not contain thimerosal. After many studies and several years, both the MMR vaccine and thimerosal were declared not to cause autism. However, because thimerosal contains a type of mercury, its use as a vaccine preservative was banned in the United States in 2001, except for tiny amounts in flu vaccines. The number of cases of autism has stayed about the same.

- **Won't so many vaccines totally overwhelm a baby's immune system?** If you're up-to-date on your vaccinations, you probably got twenty-six inoculations before you were even two years old! Some people worry that this could weaken a baby's immune system. But once you're born, you are bombarded with millions of bacteria. Your immune system imme-diately begins making antibodies to fight them. Many experts believe that babies can produce antibodies to the antigens in as many as 10,000 vaccines at one time.

No one can say that any vaccine is 100 percent safe or effective on 100 percent of the people who get it. If you have questions about a vaccine, or a lingering fear of them, you should talk to your doctor.

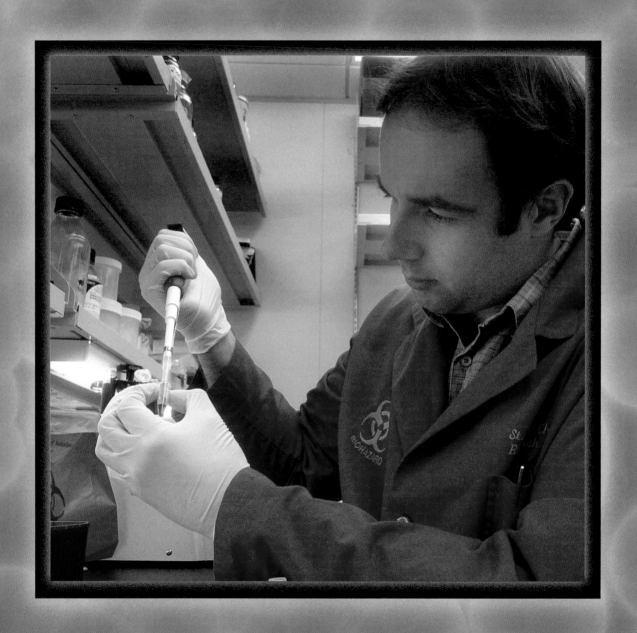

chapter 5

Vaccines of the Future

If you were born in the twenty-first century, devices such as smart phones, e-books, and instant, wireless Internet access may not amaze you. After all, you grew up with them. But you can count on researchers using technology to come up with newer, faster, smarter devices that probably will amaze you.

The same thing is happening with vaccines. Ever since Edward Jenner developed the smallpox vaccine in the eighteenth century, researchers have been working to discover newer, better, and more effective vaccines to prevent disease. The development of the vaccine

A researcher at St. Jude Children's Research Hospital in Tennessee works to develop a flu vaccine that doesn't use eggs.

for whooping cough is a good example. The first one was produced in the 1930s. It was a whole-cell vaccine. That means it contained "killed" elements of the entire pertussis microbe. In the 1940s it was combined with the diphtheria and tetanus toxoids and called the DTP vaccine.

By 1991 scientists were growing only parts of the pertussis microbe in the lab and then purifying them. This version of the vaccine for diphtheria, tetanus, and pertussis had fewer side effects than earlier ones. It is called the DTaP vaccine. It is given to children younger than seven. The Tdap vaccine came along in 2005. It is used as a booster for adolescents and adults.

Amazing New Methods

While some researchers work on improving vaccines, others experiment with new ways of making them. The DNA vaccine is one of them. Instead of using all or even some parts of a disease-causing microbe, a DNA vaccine uses its genetic material. When the genes of a microbe's antigens are used in a vaccine, some of the body's cells take up that DNA. Those cells then make antigen molecules, which cause the immune system to react. In this case the body, not the microbe, is actually producing the antigens. As one researcher put it, "The body's cells become a vaccine-making factory." The DNA vaccine could not cause disease because it contains only copies of a few genes from a microbe. It does not contain the microbe itself.

Another experimental vaccine also uses DNA. Here, a weakened virus or bacterium is combined with genetic material from another disease-causing microbe. The weakened microbe then carries those genes to the cells. Because these vaccines would mimic natural infections, they would get a strong response from the immune system.

New Vaccines for Stubborn Diseases

A major quest of researchers is to develop vaccines for diseases such as malaria and AIDS. Malaria is a mosquito-borne disease caused by a **parasite**. Malaria causes high fevers and terrible, shaking chills. It can be fatal if it is not treated. Close to 220 million cases occurred worldwide in 2010, and over 650,000 people died. Most of them were children. There are drugs to treat malaria, but the parasite is very tricky. Over time it can become resistant to the drugs. Using different technologies, scientists have developed different types of vaccines. So far all of these are still being tested, but some of the early results are very hopeful.

AIDS is a devastating disease that researchers want to conquer. It killed almost 2 million people in 2011. Every year, HIV/AIDS infects about 50,000 people in the United States. HIV is a virus that attacks and destroys the disease-fighting cells in a person's immune system. It can be treated, but researchers believe a vaccine is the best answer to it. A DNA vaccine is one type that is being tested. Some researchers believe that a vaccine could be ready by 2020.

Two vaccines help prevent cancer. The HPV vaccine can prevent some cervical cancers in women. The hepatitis B vaccine can prevent liver cancer. While researchers are trying to develop more vaccines to prevent cancer, they are also working on cancer-treatment vaccines. These vaccines would teach the immune system to recognize and attack cancer cells.

In the future, there may be vaccines that prevent drug addiction. For example, a vaccine for cocaine would make antibodies that prevent the cocaine from leaving the bloodstream. This would stop the "high" that cocaine users experience.

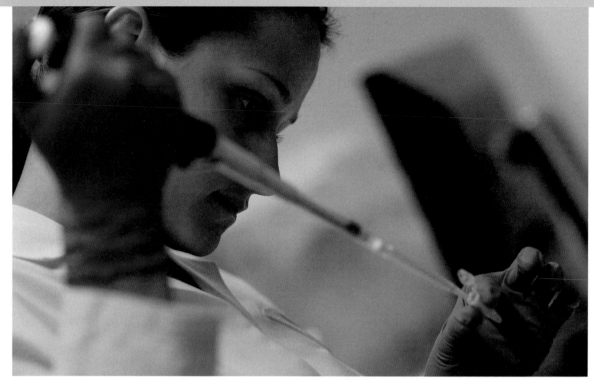

A research associate at the AIDS Vaccine Design and Development Laboratory in New York City studies new methods of cultivating a vaccine to prevent the development of this deadly disease in an infected body.

New Delivery Systems

No one likes getting a shot, which is how most vaccines are given. A lot of vaccines need to be refrigerated. That adds to the cost of the vaccines. It makes it hard to transport them, especially to remote areas. It makes it hard to store them in developing countries where electricity is sometimes hit-or-miss.

One new method being worked on is a skin patch. It would work by delivering the vaccine to the person through tiny microneedles. It would not have to be refrigerated, and it would not hurt. Vaccine skin patches are being tested for diseases such as anthrax, tetanus, and the flu.

How about an edible vaccine? Using genetic engineering, researchers are working on ways to include vaccine antigens in foods such as potatoes and bananas. When people eat the genetically engineered foods, they would get a vaccine boost. For example, if you were to eat a genetically engineered banana, you would get a dose of the pertussis vaccine. Tests have shown that this method causes the immune system to produce antibodies. One problem with edible vaccines is the difficulty of ensuring that the food contains the correct dose. Also, many people do not like the idea of eating genetically engineered food.

Other researchers are developing ways to use plants that we don't normally eat. Vaccines would be produced in a plant's leaves. The leaves would then be ground up and put into gelatin capsules. You could take them the way you take vitamins.

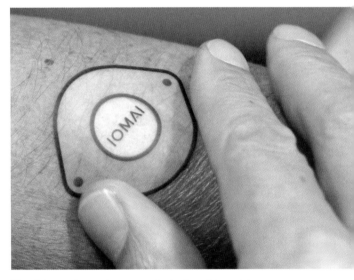

The future of vaccines may lie in the skin patch, a needle-free vaccine.

The computer program you use this year will most likely be out-of-date next year. Advances in vaccines don't happen that fast. It often takes decades of research to get to the "beta," or test, version of a vaccine. It takes more years of testing before it can be approved. New technology has helped shorten that time. A better understanding of the immune system has helped, too. It seems that new diseases will always be cropping up, but vaccines won't be far behind in catching up to them.

Glossary

anthrax A bacterial disease that can affect the skin, digestive system, and lungs. It is not spread from person to person.

antibodies Molecules produced in the immune system as a defense against bacteria and viruses.

antigens Markers on harmful microbes that cause the immune system to produce antibodies to fight the invading microbes.

attenuated Weakened; an attenuated virus is a harmless or less harmful form of a disease-causing microbe.

bacteria One-celled organisms that can cause infectious diseases.

chicken pox A viral disease that causes an itchy rash. It is spread from person to person.

contagious Capable of being transmitted by contact with an infected person or object.

diphtheria A bacterial disease that causes severe breathing problems and sometimes affects the heart and muscles. It is spread from person to person.

hepatitis A A disease caused by a virus that infects the liver. It is often transmitted by contaminated food or water.

hepatitis B A disease caused by a virus (hepatitis B virus, or HBV) that infects the liver. It can be transmitted through blood transfusion, sexual contact, or mucus in the eyes and mouth. It can cause liver cancer.

Hib disease A contagious disease that causes bacterial meningitis, an infection of the brain. It usually strikes children under five years old and can be fatal.

influenza A contagious respiratory illness caused by influenza viruses that come in many strains, changing from year to year. More commonly called the flu.

macrophages Large white blood cells that ingest, or swallow, infectious microorganisms.

measles An infectious viral disease that affects mostly children. It causes a blotchy skin rash and fever and can lead to pneumonia or deafness.

microbiology The branch of biology dealing with the structure and life of microscopic organisms.

microorganism Any organism too small to be seen without a microscope.

mumps An infectious viral disease that causes swelling of the salivary glands.

paralysis A loss or impairment of voluntary movement in a body part as a result of injury or disease of the nerves, brain, or spinal cord.

parasite An organism that lives on or inside a host (an animal or other living organism) and gets its nourishment from the host.

pertussis An infectious bacterial disease that causes a series of short, convulsive coughs often followed by a whooping sound. Often called whoooping cough.

pneumococcal disease A bacterial disease that can cause a range of infections, from mild ear infections to fatal pneumonia.

pneumonia An acute bacterial disease of the lungs that can cause fever, a cough with blood-tinged phlegm, and difficulty breathing.

polio A viral disease, usually affecting children and young adults, that invades the motor neurons of the brain and spinal cord. It can cause paralysis and death.

rabies An infectious viral disease of dogs, cats, and other animals such as raccoons and bats. It is transmitted to humans by the bite of the infected animal and is usually fatal unless it is treated.

radiation Energy in the form of high-speed particles or electromagnetic waves.

rotavirus A virus that is a major cause of infant diarrhea.

rubella A usually mild contagious viral disease causing fever, congestion, and a pink or pale red rash. If contracted by a woman during early pregnancy, it may cause mental and physical defects in the fetus. It is also called German measles.

smallpox A highly contagious viral disease that was often fatal. Those who survived had permanent pits or scars from healed pustules.

tetanus An infectious, often fatal disease caused by a bacterium that enters the body through a wound. Also known as lockjaw, it can cause paralysis and death.

virus A microbe that reproduces itself only within the cells of living hosts, which are mainly bacteria, plants, and animals

Find Out More

Books

Alter, Judy. V*accines: Innovations in Medicine.* Ann Arbor, MI: Cherry Lake Publishing, 2009.

Feinstein, Stephen. *Louis Pasteur: The Father of Microbiology.* Berkeley Heights, NJ: Enslow Publishers, 2008.

Phelan, Glen. *Killing Germs, Saving Lives: The Quest for the First Vaccines.* Washington, DC: National Geographic, 2006.

Smith, Michael Joseph, M.D., M.S.C.E, and Laurie Bouck. *The Complete Idiot's Guide to Vaccinations.* Indianapolis, IN: Alpha Books, 2010.

Websites

Centers for Disease Control
The website of the U.S. Centers for Disease Control provides information on the importance of vaccines, vaccine side effects and safety, and recent vaccine-related news.
www.cdc.gov/vaccines/

Getvaxed.org

Getvaxed.org offers information about vaccines to teens and young adults. It describes why the vaccines are important, where to get them, and what diseases they prevent.

www.getvaxed.org/

KidsHealth

KidsHealth offers information and answers to kids, teens, and parents about vaccines and immunization, as well as about eating right, exercise, and ways to lead a healthy life.

http://kidshealth.org/

National Institute of Allergy and Infectious Diseases

The website of the National Institute of Allergy and Infectious Diseases explains what vaccines are, provides information on their history, benefits, and controversies, and describes the various types of vaccines in use today.

www.niaid.nih.gov/topics/vaccines/understanding/Pages/whatVaccine.aspx

Smithsonian Museum of American History

The website of the Smithsonian Museum of American History offers an in-depth look at the history of polio in the United States, its effect on individuals, communities, and the medical community, and how it was finally conquered in the United States.

www.americanhistory.si.edu/polio/americanepi/index.htm

Index

Page numbers in **boldface** are illustrations.

About the Author

Carol Ellis enjoys writing books for young people. She has written several titles in various series, including Great Pets, Endangered!, and Martial Arts in Action. Ms. Ellis lives in New York State's Hudson River Valley.